ILEOSTOMY DIET AND MEAL PLAN SIMPLIFIED

Ileostomy Life Saver

A Culinary Expedition For A Healthy Life After Surgery

DR. SOFIA SILAS

Table of Contents

CHAPTER ONE

Introduction

Living with an ileostomy may be a difficult transition for those who have had surgery for inflammatory bowel disease, colorectal cancer, or other gastrointestinal problems. An ileostomy is the surgical construction of a stoma in the abdomen through which waste is transferred to an external pouch.

This technique may significantly enhance the quality of life for those with certain medical issues, but it also requires adaptation and lifestyle modifications. In this conversation, we will look at what it means to live with an ileostomy, including post-surgery preparation, nutritional concerns, and ideas for constructing a balanced meal plan to promote general health and well-being.

Understanding Ileostomy

An ileostomy is a surgical technique in which the ileum, or bottom section of the small intestine, is diverted via an incision in the abdominal wall.

This causes the formation of a stoma, which protrudes slightly from the belly and is where waste materials depart the body. The stoma is usually red or pink in hue and lacks nerve endings, making it painless to touch.

Following surgery, waste products such as feces and mucus flow through the stoma and are collected in a pouch worn outside the body. Depending on the kind of ileostomy, the stool may be liquid or semi-formed since the colon, which absorbs water from waste, is bypassed.

Living with an ileostomy necessitates knowing how to care for the stoma and pouch, which includes adequate cleanliness, changing the pouch as needed, and managing any issues including skin irritation or leaking. While these chores may seem onerous at first, many people discover that with time and experience, they become ordinary aspects of their daily lives.

Preparing For Life Following Surgery

Before having ileostomy surgery, you should have a clear awareness of what to anticipate both before and after the process. This may include speaking with healthcare experts, attending pre-operative education classes, and connecting with support groups or others who have lived with an ileostomy.

Patients may suffer soreness, exhaustion, and changes in bowel function in the days after surgery as their bodies adapt to the procedure. During this period, it is critical to adhere to healthcare specialists' advice for pain management, activity level, and nutritional changes.

As recuperation develops, people may gradually resume typical activities including work, exercise, and socializing. However, it may take some time to properly adapt to life with an ileostomy, both physically and mentally. Obtaining assistance from loved ones, healthcare experts, and peer support groups may be quite beneficial during this transition phase.

Nutritional Needs With An Ileostomy

Maintaining sufficient nourishment is critical for general health and well-being, particularly for those with an ileostomy. People with ileostomies are at risk for dehydration, electrolyte imbalances, and vitamin deficiencies if their food intake is not properly regulated because of the bypassing of the colon, which plays an important role in water and electrolyte absorption.

Fluid and electrolyte balance is a major problem for those who have had an ileostomy. Because the colon absorbs water and electrolytes from waste, those who have an ileostomy may suffer greater fluid loss via the stoma.

Staying well-hydrated requires consuming enough fluids throughout the day, including water, electrolyte-rich drinks, and, if required, oral rehydration treatments.

In addition to water, it is important to consume enough dietary fiber. Although the colon is bypassed with an ileostomy, some people may still have problems with stool consistency and bowel function. Soluble fiber from cereals, fruits, and vegetables may be introduced gradually to help bulk up stool and control bowel motions.

CHAPTER TWO

Creating A Balanced Meal Plan

When preparing meals with an ileostomy, it is critical to prioritize nutrient-dense foods that include a balance of carbs, protein, fat, vitamins, and minerals. This may assist in maintaining general health and energy levels while reducing the danger of dietary shortages.

Aim to incorporate a variety of foods from each dietary category, including:

1. Lean proteins include chicken, fish, eggs, tofu, and lentils.

2. Whole grains include brown rice, quinoa, whole wheat bread, and oats.

3. Consume raw and cooked fruits and vegetables for vitamin, mineral, and fiber benefits.

4. Consume healthy fats like nuts, seeds, avocados, and olive oil.

It may be beneficial to eat smaller, more frequent meals throughout the day rather than three big meals, as this may help avoid digestive overload and reduce the risk of ostomy-related problems such as gas, bloating, and diarrhea.

It is also critical to watch portion sizes and chew meals completely to improve digestion and avoid obstructions in the digestive tract. Some people may need to avoid items that are difficult to digest or irritate their stomas, such as tough meats, fibrous vegetables, and high-fiber cereals.

In conclusion, living with an ileostomy necessitates changes in both lifestyle and nutritional habits. Individuals who grasp the fundamentals of ileostomy care, prepare for life after surgery, and pay attention to dietary requirements may effectively traverse the obstacles of living with an ileostomy and have a meaningful and healthy life.

Grocery shopping guidelines are necessary for anybody wanting to maintain a healthy and balanced diet, but it is especially important for those with special dietary requirements, such as those with an ileostomy, to make educated decisions.

Navigating the aisles with a focus on meals that are both healthy and soothing on the digestive system may significantly enhance one's quality of life. Here are some tips for efficient and productive supermarket shopping:

First and foremost, make a strategy ahead of time. Before you go shopping, develop a list of ileostomy-friendly meals for the week. This might help you avoid impulsive purchases and make sure you have everything you need to cook delicious meals and snacks.

When purchasing vegetables, choose ones that are simple to digest and unlikely to cause discomfort. This might include fruits like bananas, applesauce, and peeled, seedless kinds, as well as veggies like cooked carrots, zucchini, and spinach. Avoiding high-fiber meals, such as fresh fruits and vegetables, helps reduce the chance of blockages and discomfort.

In the meat and fish department, go for lean protein choices that are easy on the stomach. Skinless chicken, fish, and soft cuts of beef or hog are also good possibilities. Consider including plant-based proteins in your diet, such as tofu, tempeh, or lentils, for extra variety and nutritional value.

When shopping for pantry basics, emphasize foods with minimal added sugars, salt, and artificial additives. Choose whole grains like brown rice, quinoa, and oats, as well as unprocessed carbs like sweet potatoes and whole-grain bread or pasta. Look for canned foods with no added salt, and choose low-fat or fat-free dairy items such as yogurt and cheese.

When making meals for people with ileostomies, it's important to use cooking methods that are easy on the digestive system. Steaming, boiling, baking, and poaching are all wonderful ways to maintain moisture and taste without adding too much fat or creating discomfort.

Avoid frying or grilling meals at high heat since these procedures might produce chemicals that are difficult to digest.

Building taste without irritating is another crucial issue when cooking for those with ileostomies. Herbs and spices may be used extensively to improve the flavor of foods without adding too much salt or fat.

Experiment using fresh herbs like parsley, basil, and cilantro, as well as spices like ginger, turmeric, and cinnamon, to add depth and complexity to your recipes.

Hydration And Fluid Consumption

Hydration and fluid consumption are critical components of sustaining general health and well-being, particularly for those with ileostomy.

Drink lots of water throughout the day to avoid dehydration and to regulate bowel function. In addition to water, try to include hydrating foods such as cucumbers, melons, and soups or broths in your diet to increase fluid consumption.

Snack alternatives for rapid energy might help you stay fuelled and satisfied between meals while avoiding pain or aggravation. Choose nutrient-dense foods such as nuts and seeds, dried fruit, yogurt, or whole-grain crackers with hummus.

Smoothies created with protein-rich ingredients such as Greek yogurt, nut butter, and leafy greens may also be an easy and invigorating snack option.

To summarize, grocery shopping for someone with an ileostomy requires careful consideration of dietary requirements and preferences. It is feasible to prepare tasty and nutritious meals that promote overall health and well-being by preparing ahead of time, selecting foods that are easy on the stomach, and combining distinctive cooking methods. Remember to remain hydrated and have a range of nutrient-dense foods available for rapid energy throughout the day.

Dining Out With Confidence

Dining out with an ileostomy might provide particular complications. However, with the appropriate strategy, you may dine out with confidence and satisfaction. One important factor is to plan.

Researching restaurant menus online might help you find selections that meet your dietary requirements. Furthermore, contacting the restaurant ahead of time to discuss your needs might make your eating experience go more smoothly.

CHAPTER THREE
Dealing With Digestive Challenges

Individuals with an ileostomy have a variety of digestive difficulties. These problems may include diarrhea, gas, or bloating. To treat these symptoms, you must pay attention to your diet and identify trigger foods that might aggravate digestive problems.

Keeping a food diary might help you understand how various meals influence your digestive system. Furthermore, keeping hydrated and eating smaller, more frequent meals might help digestion and relieve discomfort.

Managing Weight Change

Weight fluctuations are a concern for many people with ileostomies, especially if they have malabsorption or appetite changes.

To properly control weight, concentrate on nutrient-dense meals that include necessary vitamins and minerals. Eating lean meats, fruits, vegetables, and whole grains may help you maintain a healthy weight. Regular exercise may also help you manage your weight and improve your general health.

Exploring Dietary Supplements

Individuals with an ileostomy might benefit from dietary supplements to help them maintain their overall health and wellness.

However, it is critical to contact a healthcare practitioner before beginning any new supplements, since they may mix with drugs or aggravate pre-existing health concerns. Multivitamins, probiotics, and iron supplements are all examples of potentially useful supplements. Working with a licensed dietitian may help you customize a supplement program to match your specific nutritional requirements.

Social Implications Of Dining With An Ileostomy

Dining out with friends and family may be a fun and sociable activity. However, it is normal to feel self-conscious while eating with an ileostomy.

One approach for dealing with these sentiments is to concentrate on the company rather than the meal. Engaging in meaningful discussion and enjoying the social side of meals might assist in moving the emphasis away from any ileostomy-related anxieties. Furthermore, selecting restaurants with private or accessible toilets may bring an extra piece of mind while eating out.

To summarize, addressing the problems of dining with an ileostomy involves careful preparation, attentive eating, and an emphasis on overall health and well-being.

Individuals with an ileostomy may dine out confidently and enjoyably by making proactive efforts to treat digestive difficulties, control weight fluctuations, investigate nutritional supplements, and embrace the social elements of eating. Dining out can be a rewarding event for everyone involved if the correct methods and assistance are used.

CHAPTER FOUR

Physical Activity And Nutrition

Maintaining a healthy lifestyle requires a harmonious mix of physical activity and a good diet. These two components are inextricably intertwined, with each playing an important role in fostering general health and vitality.

Physical exercise is required to maintain a healthy body weight, improve cardiovascular health, and increase muscular strength and flexibility. Regular exercise not only burns calories, but also improves mood, decreases stress, and promotes healthier sleep habits. A well-rounded fitness plan includes a range of activities such as aerobic workouts, weight training, and flexibility exercises.

To get the most advantages from physical exercise, it must be combined with an appropriate diet. Fueling the body with the correct nutrients before and after exercise may help improve performance, recuperation, and muscular development.

A well-balanced diet rich in whole foods, such as fruits, vegetables, lean meats, and whole grains, has the nutrients required to maintain energy levels and support general health.

Proper diet is important for both physical and mental wellbeing. According to research, some nutrients, such as omega-3 fatty acids, vitamins B and D, and antioxidants, have an important role in brain function and mood regulation. A diet high in these nutrients may help lower the risk of depression, anxiety, and cognitive impairment.

Mental Health And Nutrition

The link between mental health and diet emphasizes the need to take a comprehensive approach to well-being. Nutritional deficits have a detrimental influence on mood, cognitive function, and general mental well-being. In contrast, eating a well-balanced diet that promotes brain function may help relieve stress, anxiety, and depression.

Certain nutrients have been shown to have mood-enhancing qualities. Omega-3 fatty acids, present in fatty fish such as salmon and walnuts, are important for brain function and have been related to a lower incidence of depression. Similarly, antioxidant-rich foods like berries, leafy greens, and dark chocolate aid in the fight against oxidative stress and inflammation, all of which have been linked to mood problems.

Maintaining steady blood sugar levels is also beneficial to mental wellness. Consuming complex carbs such as whole grains, legumes, and vegetables offers a consistent supply of energy for the brain, reducing mood and energy changes. Incorporating lean proteins and healthy fats into meals also promotes satiety and regulates blood sugar levels.

Furthermore, hydration is important for cognitive function

and mood management. Dehydration may decrease focus, increase tiredness, and lower mood. Staying hydrated by drinking water throughout the day is critical for proper brain function and mental health.

Travel Tips For Ileostomy Patients

Traveling with an ileostomy might provide particular complications. However, with careful planning and preparation, it is feasible to enjoy a vacation while successfully managing an ileostomy.

First and foremost, bring a enough quantity of ostomy

supplies such as pouches, adhesives, and cleaning wipes. Depending on the length of the journey and the availability of medical supplies at the destination, it may be essential to take additional supplies to guarantee continuity of treatment.

When traveling, it is best to keep ostomy equipment in carry-on baggage to avoid loss or damage. It is also beneficial to alert airport security of the presence of medical supplies to speed up the screening procedure.

Researching medical facilities at the location and being acquainted with local healthcare options may bring peace of mind in the event of a medical emergency or supply shortage.

Maintaining a healthy diet while traveling is critical for ileostomy patients to avoid issues like dehydration and obstructions. Avoiding meals that might cause ostomy output to become overly thick or watery, such as high-fiber or spicy foods, can aid in maintaining good ostomy performance.

Staying hydrated is also important, particularly while traveling to hot or humid areas.

Drinking lots of water and avoiding excessive alcohol and caffeine use might help you stay hydrated and keep your electrolytes balanced.

CHAPTER FIVE

Support Systems And Resources

Living with a chronic disease or making major lifestyle changes may be difficult, but having a solid support system in place can make a huge difference. Friends, family, support groups, and healthcare experts may all give helpful emotional support and practical assistance.

Individuals with specialized health issues, such as ostomy support groups, benefit from a safe and understanding atmosphere in which to discuss difficulties, exchange ideas and resources, and get encouragement from others who have had similar experiences.

In addition to peer support, tools like online forums, instructional materials, and counseling services may help you navigate the physical, emotional, and logistical elements of living with a chronic disease.

Nurses, nutritionists, and mental health specialists all play important roles in providing specialized treatment and advice based on individual requirements. A collaborative connection with healthcare professionals promotes open communication and ensures that patients get comprehensive treatment that meets their specific issues and aspirations.

Conclusion

To summarize, the interdependence of physical exercise, diet, mental health, and support networks emphasizes the significance of a comprehensive approach to well-being. A healthy lifestyle includes frequent physical exercise, a well-balanced diet, and a focus on mental health.

Individuals with chronic diseases, such as an ileostomy, need careful planning and preparation to provide continuity of treatment when traveling. Building a solid support system and gaining access to services and healthcare specialists may be quite beneficial while navigating the obstacles of chronic disease.

Individuals may improve their well-being and live life to the fullest by prioritizing self-care, getting help when required, and adopting a proactive attitude to health and wellbeing, regardless of any barriers they may encounter.